DETOXIFY: THE CANCER-FIGHTING JUICE GUIDE

DETOXIFY YOUR BODY AND BOOST YOUR HEALTH

Author: K. Griffiths MSN Ed FNP-C

Copyright © 2020 Griffiths

TABLE OF CONTENTS

Chapter 1: Understanding Cancer and Juicing for Detoxification

The Link Between Cancer and Toxins

Cancer is a complex disease that can be caused by a variety of factors, including genetics, lifestyle choices, and environmental toxins. In recent years, there has been growing evidence to suggest that exposure to certain toxins may play a significant role in the development of cancer. This subchapter will explore the link between cancer and toxins, and how juicing can help to detoxify the body and reduce the risk of cancer.

Toxins are substances that can cause harm to the body, and they are found in a wide range of everyday products, from cleaning supplies to pesticides to personal care products. When these toxins are absorbed into the body, they can disrupt normal cellular function and increase the risk of developing cancer. Studies have shown that certain toxins, such as benzene and asbestos, are known carcinogens and can significantly increase the risk of developing cancer.

One of the key benefits of juicing is that it can help to detoxify the body and eliminate harmful toxins. By consuming a diet rich in fruits and vegetables, which are high in antioxidants and other nutrients, you can help to support the body's natural detoxification processes and reduce the burden of toxins on the body. Juicing can also help to support the liver, which is responsible for filtering out toxins and waste products from the body.

In addition to juicing, there are a number of other steps you can take to reduce your exposure to toxins and lower your risk of cancer. This includes choosing organic produce whenever possible, avoiding processed foods and drinks that are high in additives and preservatives, and using natural cleaning and personal care products. By making these simple changes to your lifestyle, you can help to protect your body from harmful toxins and reduce your risk of developing cancer.

In conclusion, the link between cancer and toxins is a complex and multifaceted issue, but by taking steps to detoxify the body and reduce exposure to harmful substances, you can help to lower your risk of developing cancer. Juicing is a powerful tool for detoxifying the body and supporting overall health, and can be an important part of a comprehensive cancer-fighting strategy. By incorporating juicing into your daily routine and making other healthy lifestyle choices, you can help to protect your body from the harmful effects of toxins and boost your overall health and well-being.

Benefits of Juicing for Detoxification

Juicing has gained popularity in recent years as a way to detoxify the body and improve overall health. For cancer patients, incorporating fresh juices into their diet can have numerous benefits. One of the key advantages of juicing for detoxification is that it allows the body to easily absorb essential nutrients from fruits and vegetables. This is especially important for cancer patients, as their bodies may have difficulty processing solid foods or extracting nutrients from them.

Another benefit of juicing for detoxification is that it can help to alkalize the body. Cancer cells thrive in an acidic environment, so by consuming alkaline-rich juices, patients can create a more hostile environment for cancer cells to grow. Additionally, juicing can help to reduce inflammation in the body, which is a common side effect of cancer and its treatments. By including anti-inflammatory ingredients like turmeric, ginger, and leafy greens in their juices, cancer patients can help to alleviate pain and discomfort.

Juicing for detoxification can also support the body's natural detoxification processes. The liver, kidneys, and other organs work tirelessly to rid the body of toxins, but they can become overwhelmed, especially in cancer patients. By providing the body with an abundance of nutrients in an easily digestible form, juicing can help to support these organs and enhance their detoxification capabilities. This can lead to improved energy levels, clearer skin, and a stronger immune system.

In addition to supporting detoxification, juicing can also help cancer patients to maintain a healthy weight. Many cancer treatments can cause weight loss or weight gain, both of which can have negative impacts on overall health. Juicing allows patients to control their calorie intake while still ensuring they are receiving essential nutrients. By incorporating a variety of fruits and vegetables into their juices, cancer patients can maintain a healthy weight and support their body's healing process.

Overall, juicing for detoxification can be a valuable tool for cancer patients looking to improve their health and well-being. By incorporating fresh juices into their diet, patients can support their body's natural detoxification processes, reduce inflammation, and maintain a healthy weight. Juicing can also provide cancer patients with a convenient and delicious way to consume essential nutrients and support their overall health during their cancer journey.

How Juicing Can Support Cancer Treatment

Cancer treatment can be a challenging journey, both physically and emotionally. Alongside traditional medical treatments, many cancer patients are turning to alternative therapies to support their bodies during this difficult time. Juicing has gained popularity as a natural way to detoxify the body and boost overall health, making it a valuable tool for cancer patients looking to support their treatment.

Juicing is a powerful way to flood the body with essential nutrients that can help strengthen the immune system and support the body's natural detoxification processes. Cancer treatments such as chemotherapy and radiation can take a toll on the body, causing fatigue, nausea, and a weakened immune system. By incorporating fresh, nutrient-dense juices into their diets, cancer patients can give their bodies the support they need to heal and recover.

One of the key benefits of juicing for cancer patients is the ability to easily consume a large quantity of fruits and vegetables in a single serving. Juicing allows nutrients to be rapidly absorbed by the body, providing a quick and easy way to get essential vitamins, minerals, and antioxidants.

These nutrients can help support the body's natural detoxification pathways, reduce inflammation, and boost overall health.

Certain fruits and vegetables have been shown to have cancer-fighting properties, making them ideal choices for juicing. Ingredients such as leafy greens, berries, turmeric, and ginger are rich in antioxidants and anti-inflammatory compounds that can help protect cells from damage and support the body's natural defenses against cancer. By incorporating these ingredients into their juicing routines, cancer patients can give their bodies an extra boost of support during treatment.

Overall, juicing can be a valuable tool for cancer patients looking to support their bodies during treatment. By providing a quick and easy way to consume essential nutrients, juicing can help strengthen the immune system, support detoxification, and boost overall health. With the guidance of a healthcare provider or nutritionist, cancer patients can safely incorporate juicing into their treatment plans to help optimize their health and well-being.

Chapter 2: The Best Cancer-Fighting Ingredients for Juicing

Cruciferous Vegetables

Cruciferous vegetables are a powerhouse of nutrients that have been shown to have numerous health benefits, especially for cancer patients undergoing treatment. These vegetables, which include broccoli, cauliflower, kale, and Brussels sprouts, are rich in antioxidants, vitamins, and minerals that can help detoxify the body and boost overall health. Juicing these vegetables is an excellent way to incorporate them into your diet and reap their many benefits.

One of the key components of cruciferous vegetables is their high levels of phytochemicals, which are compounds that have been shown to have anti-cancer properties. These phytochemicals work to neutralize free radicals in the body, which can damage cells and lead to the development of cancer. By incorporating cruciferous vegetables into your juicing routine, you can help protect your cells from this damage and reduce your risk of developing cancer.

In addition to their cancer-fighting properties, cruciferous vegetables are also rich in fiber, which is essential for maintaining a healthy digestive system. Fiber helps to regulate digestion, prevent constipation, and promote the growth of beneficial bacteria in the gut. By juicing cruciferous vegetables, you can easily increase your fiber intake and support your digestive health, which is especially important for cancer patients undergoing treatment.

Furthermore, cruciferous vegetables are a great source of vitamins A, C, and K, as well as minerals like potassium and calcium. These nutrients are essential for maintaining a strong immune system, supporting bone health, and promoting overall well-being. By juicing cruciferous vegetables, you can easily incorporate these vital nutrients into your diet and give your body the support it needs to fight off illness and stay healthy during cancer treatment.

Overall, incorporating cruciferous vegetables into your juicing routine is a simple and effective way to boost your health and support your body during cancer treatment. These vegetables are packed with essential nutrients and phytochemicals that can help detoxify your body, reduce inflammation, and protect your cells from damage. Whether you juice them on their own or combine them with other fruits and vegetables, cruciferous vegetables are a valuable addition to any cancer-fighting juicing regimen.

Berries

Berries are an essential ingredient in any cancer-fighting juicing regimen. These tiny fruits are packed with antioxidants and phytochemicals that have been shown to help prevent and fight cancer. Berries like blueberries, strawberries, raspberries, and blackberries are not only delicious but also incredibly nutritious. They are rich in vitamins, minerals, and fiber, making them the perfect addition to any detoxifying juice.

One of the key benefits of incorporating berries into your juicing routine is their high antioxidant content. Antioxidants help to neutralize free radicals in the body, which can cause cell damage and lead to cancer. Berries are particularly rich in antioxidants like vitamin C and ellagic acid, which have been linked to a reduced risk of cancer. By including a variety of berries in your juices, you can help to boost your body's natural defenses against cancer.

In addition to their antioxidant properties, berries are also a great source of fiber. Fiber is important for detoxifying the body and promoting healthy digestion. Berries contain both soluble and insoluble fiber, which can help to regulate blood sugar levels, lower cholesterol, and promote a healthy gut microbiome. By regularly consuming berry juices, you can support your body's natural detoxification processes and improve overall health.

When juicing with berries, it's important to choose organic varieties whenever possible. Conventionally grown berries can be high in pesticides and other harmful chemicals, which can negate the health benefits of these fruits. Look for organic berries at your local farmers' market or natural foods store to ensure that you are getting the purest and most nutritious ingredients for your juices.

In conclusion, berries are a powerhouse ingredient for anyone looking to detoxify their body and boost their health, especially cancer patients. Their antioxidant-rich, fiber-packed properties make them a valuable addition to any juicing regimen. By incorporating a variety of berries into your juices on a regular basis, you can help to support your body's natural detoxification processes and strengthen your defenses against cancer. So go ahead and start juicing with berries today for a delicious and nutritious way to fight cancer and improve your overall well-being.

Leafy Greens

Leafy greens are a crucial component of any cancer-fighting juicing regimen. Packed with essential vitamins, minerals, and antioxidants, these vegetables provide a powerful defense against cancer cells and help to detoxify the body from harmful toxins. From spinach and kale to arugula and Swiss chard, leafy greens offer a wide range of health benefits that can support cancer patients on their journey to recovery.

One of the key nutrients found in leafy greens is chlorophyll, which has been shown to have anti-cancer properties. Chlorophyll helps to neutralize carcinogens in the body and promote the elimination of toxins through the liver and kidneys. By incorporating leafy greens into your daily juicing routine, you can boost your body's natural detoxification processes and reduce your risk of developing cancer.

In addition to chlorophyll, leafy greens are also rich in other cancer-fighting compounds such as sulforaphane, indole-3-carbinol, and quercetin. These phytochemicals work together to inhibit the growth of cancer cells, reduce inflammation, and protect against DNA damage. By juicing a variety of leafy greens, you can ensure that you are getting a diverse array of cancer-fighting nutrients that can help to support your body's immune system and promote overall wellness.

When juicing leafy greens, it is important to choose organic produce whenever possible to avoid exposure to pesticides and other harmful chemicals. Washing your greens thoroughly before juicing can also help to remove any residue that may be present on the surface of the vegetables. By incorporating a variety of leafy greens into your juicing recipes, you can create delicious and nutritious drinks that support your body's natural detoxification processes and help to boost your overall health.

In conclusion, leafy greens are an essential component of any cancer-fighting juicing regimen. Packed with vitamins, minerals, and antioxidants, these vegetables offer a wide range of health benefits that can help to detoxify the body and reduce the risk of developing cancer. By juicing a variety of leafy greens on a regular basis, you can support your body's natural detoxification processes, boost your immune system, and improve your overall health and well-being.

Turmeric

Turmeric is a powerful spice that has gained a lot of attention in recent years for its incredible health benefits, particularly in relation to cancer. This bright yellow spice has been used for centuries in traditional medicine for its anti-inflammatory and antioxidant properties. In recent years, scientists have discovered that turmeric contains a compound called curcumin, which has been shown to have powerful anti-cancer properties.

Studies have shown that curcumin can help to prevent the growth and spread of cancer cells, as well as reduce inflammation in the body. In fact, some studies have shown that curcumin may be as effective as certain chemotherapy drugs in treating cancer. This makes turmeric a valuable addition to any cancer-fighting juicing regimen.

When juicing for detoxifying the body in cancer patients, it is important to include turmeric in your recipes. Turmeric can help to cleanse the liver, which is essential for detoxifying the body and removing toxins that can contribute to the development of cancer. Additionally, turmeric can help to reduce inflammation in the body, which is important for supporting the immune system and preventing the growth and spread of cancer cells.

One easy way to incorporate turmeric into your juicing routine is to add a small piece of fresh turmeric root to your juice recipes. You can also use ground turmeric powder if fresh turmeric is not available. Turmeric pairs well with fruits like pineapple, mango, and orange, as well as vegetables like carrots and beets. Experiment with different combinations to find a recipe that you enjoy and that supports your health goals.

In conclusion, turmeric is a powerful spice that can help to detoxify the body and boost your health, particularly when juicing for cancer patients. By including turmeric in your juicing recipes, you can take advantage of its anti-cancer properties and support your body in fighting off disease. So next time you fire up your juicer, be sure to add a little turmeric for a delicious and health-boosting kick!

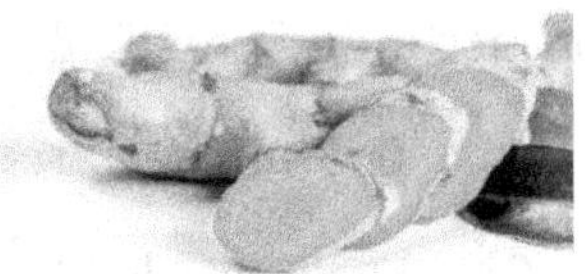

Ginger

Ginger has long been recognized for its powerful healing properties, especially when it comes to detoxifying the body and boosting overall health. This spicy root has been used for centuries in traditional medicine to treat a variety of ailments, including nausea, inflammation, and digestive issues. In recent years, ginger has gained popularity in the world of juicing as a key ingredient in cancer-fighting recipes.

One of the main reasons ginger is so beneficial for cancer patients is its ability to reduce inflammation in the body. Chronic inflammation has been linked to the development and progression of cancer, so it is crucial to incorporate anti-inflammatory foods like ginger into your diet. Juicing fresh ginger root along with other fruits and vegetables can help to reduce inflammation and support your body's natural detoxification processes.

In addition to its anti-inflammatory properties, ginger is also a powerful antioxidant. Antioxidants help to neutralize free radicals in the body, which can damage cells and contribute to the development of cancer. By juicing ginger along with other antioxidant-rich ingredients like berries and leafy greens, you can help to protect your cells from oxidative stress and support your body's ability to fight off cancer.

Ginger is also known for its ability to soothe nausea, which can be a common side effect of cancer treatment. Juicing fresh ginger root with ingredients like apples and carrots can help to calm an upset stomach and improve digestion. This can be especially helpful for cancer patients who may be experiencing digestive issues as a result of their treatment.

Overall, ginger is a versatile and powerful ingredient that can play a key role in a cancer-fighting juicing regimen. Whether you are looking to reduce inflammation, boost your body's detoxification processes, or soothe nausea, ginger can provide a natural solution. By incorporating fresh ginger root into your juicing routine, you can support your body's fight against cancer and improve your overall health and well-being.

Sour Sop

Sour sop, also known as graviola, is a tropical fruit that has gained popularity in recent years for its potential cancer-fighting properties. This unique fruit is rich in antioxidants, vitamins, and minerals that can help detoxify the body and boost overall health. Juicing sour sop is a convenient and delicious way to incorporate this powerful fruit into your diet, especially for cancer patients looking to support their treatment plan.

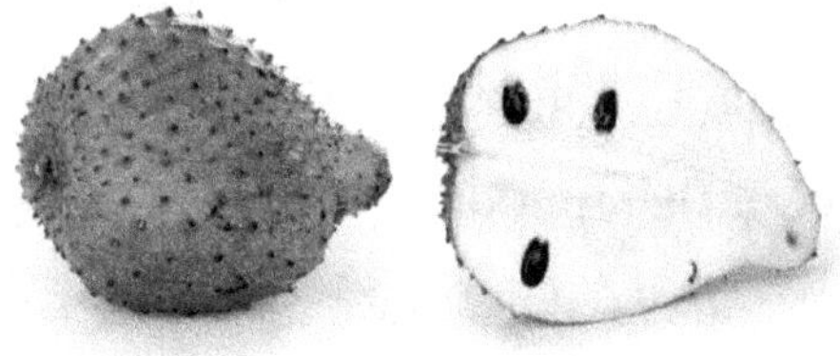

When juicing sour sop, it is important to use ripe fruit for the best flavor and nutritional benefits. The flesh of the fruit is soft and creamy, making it easy to juice and blend with other fruits and vegetables. Adding sour sop juice to your daily routine can help cleanse the body of toxins and promote healthy cell function, which is crucial for cancer patients undergoing treatment.

Research has shown that sour sop contains compounds that may help inhibit the growth of cancer cells and reduce inflammation in the body. These properties make sour sop an ideal addition to a detoxifying juice regimen for cancer patients. Juicing sour sop with other anti-inflammatory ingredients like ginger, turmeric, and leafy greens can further enhance its cancer-fighting potential.

In addition to its cancer-fighting properties, sour sop is also a good source of fiber, which can help support digestion and maintain a healthy gut microbiome. This is important for cancer patients, as chemotherapy and other treatments can often disrupt the digestive system. Juicing sour sop can help alleviate symptoms like bloating, constipation, and indigestion, making it easier for patients to maintain a balanced and nutritious diet.

Overall, incorporating sour sop juice into your daily routine can help detoxify the body, boost your immune system, and support your overall health during cancer treatment. Whether you are looking to prevent cancer or support your body through treatment, juicing sour sop is a delicious and effective way to nourish your body from the inside out.

Broccoli

Broccoli is often hailed as a superfood when it comes to fighting cancer due to its high levels of antioxidants and other beneficial compounds. When it comes to juicing for detoxifying the body in cancer patients, broccoli should definitely be a staple ingredient in your recipes.

One of the key components in broccoli that makes it so effective in fighting cancer is sulforaphane. This powerful compound has been shown to help detoxify the body by enhancing the liver's ability to remove carcinogens and other harmful substances. Including broccoli in your juicing routine can help support your body's natural detoxification processes and reduce the risk of cancer development.

In addition to its detoxifying properties, broccoli is also packed with vitamins and minerals that can help boost your overall health. It is rich in vitamin C, which can help strengthen the immune system and reduce inflammation in the body. Broccoli also contains fiber, which can aid in digestion and promote gut health, another important factor in cancer prevention and treatment.

When juicing broccoli, it is important to use fresh, organic produce to ensure that you are getting the maximum benefits. You can juice broccoli on its own or combine it with other cancer-fighting ingredients like kale, spinach, and turmeric for a powerful detoxifying blend. Experiment with different recipes to find combinations that you enjoy and that provide you with the most health benefits.

Overall, incorporating broccoli into your juicing routine can be a simple yet effective way to support your body's natural detoxification processes and boost your overall health. Whether you are a cancer patient or simply looking to prevent disease, juicing with broccoli can be a delicious and nutritious addition to your daily routine.

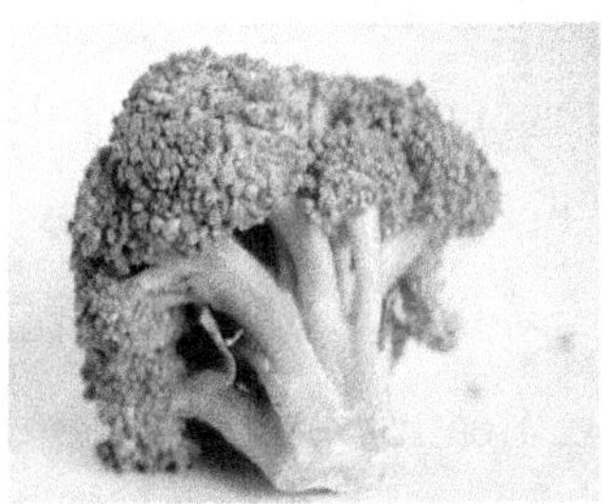

Chapter 3: Juicing Recipes for Detoxification and Health Boosting

Green Detox Juice

Green detox juice is a powerful tool in the fight against cancer. Packed with essential nutrients and antioxidants, this juice can help detoxify the body and boost overall health. By incorporating green detox juice into your daily routine, you can support your body's natural detoxification processes and give your immune system a much-needed boost.

To make green detox juice, you will need a variety of green vegetables such as kale, spinach, and celery. These vegetables are rich in vitamins, minerals, and antioxidants that can help support your body's detoxification processes. You can also add in other ingredients such as cucumber, parsley, and lemon to enhance the flavor and nutrient content of your juice.

One of the key benefits of green detox juice is its ability to help alkalize the body. Cancer cells thrive in an acidic environment, so by alkalizing your body with green detox juice, you can create a less hospitable environment for cancer to grow. Additionally, the antioxidants in green detox juice can help neutralize harmful free radicals that can damage cells and contribute to the development of cancer.

Incorporating green detox juice into your daily routine is a simple and effective way to support your body's natural detoxification processes. By providing your body with a steady supply of essential nutrients and antioxidants, you can help boost your immune system and reduce your risk of developing cancer. Whether you are currently fighting cancer or looking to prevent it in the future, green detox juice can be a valuable addition to your overall health and wellness routine.

In conclusion, green detox juice is a powerful tool for detoxifying the body and boosting overall health. By incorporating this nutrient-rich juice into your daily routine, you can support your body's natural detoxification processes and give your immune system a much-needed boost. Whether you are currently battling cancer or looking to prevent it in the future, green detox juice can be a valuable addition to your health and wellness arsenal.

Berry Blast Juice

Berry Blast Juice is a delicious and nutritious juice that can be a powerful weapon in the fight against cancer. Made with a combination of antioxidant-rich berries, this juice is packed with vitamins, minerals, and phytonutrients that can help detoxify the body and boost overall health.

One of the key ingredients in Berry Blast Juice is blueberries, which are known for their high levels of antioxidants. Antioxidants help to neutralize harmful free radicals in the body, which can reduce inflammation and protect cells from damage. This can be especially beneficial for cancer patients, as inflammation and oxidative stress are often associated with the development and progression of cancer.

Another important ingredient in Berry Blast Juice is strawberries, which are rich in vitamin C and other immune-boosting nutrients. Vitamin C is essential for a healthy immune system, and can help the body fight off infections and illnesses. Additionally, strawberries contain ellagic acid, a compound that has been shown to have anti-cancer properties.

Raspberries and blackberries are also featured in Berry Blast Juice, providing a burst of flavor and even more cancer-fighting benefits. These berries are rich in fiber, which can help to support healthy digestion and eliminate toxins from the body. They also contain a variety of vitamins and minerals that are essential for overall health and well-being.

Incorporating Berry Blast Juice into your daily routine can be a simple and delicious way to support your body's natural detoxification processes and boost your overall health. Whether you are currently undergoing cancer treatment or simply looking to improve your overall well-being, this juice can be a powerful ally in the fight against cancer. So why not give it a try and enjoy a refreshing and nutritious glass of Berry Blast Juice today?

Anti-Inflammatory Turmeric Juice

Turmeric has long been revered for its anti-inflammatory properties, making it a powerful ingredient in the fight against cancer. One of the best ways to incorporate turmeric into your diet is by juicing it. This Anti-Inflammatory Turmeric Juice recipe is not only delicious but also packed with nutrients that can help detoxify your body and boost your overall health.

To make this juice, you will need a few simple ingredients: fresh turmeric root, carrots, oranges, ginger, and a dash of black pepper. Turmeric contains a compound called curcumin, which has been shown to have powerful anti-inflammatory effects. By combining it with other immune-boosting ingredients like ginger and vitamin C-rich oranges, you can create a potent juice that will help your body fight off cancer cells and reduce inflammation.

When juicing turmeric, it is important to note that the root can stain your hands and countertops. To prevent this, wear gloves while handling the turmeric and be sure to clean your juicer thoroughly after making the juice. The vibrant orange color of this juice is a clear indication of its high antioxidant content, which can help protect your cells from damage and support your body's natural detoxification processes.

Drinking this Anti-Inflammatory Turmeric Juice regularly can help reduce inflammation in the body, which is a key factor in the development and progression of cancer. In addition to its anti-inflammatory properties, turmeric has also been shown to inhibit the growth of cancer cells and promote the death of existing cancer cells. By incorporating this juice into your daily routine, you can give your body a powerful tool for fighting off cancer and boosting your overall health.

Overall, juicing for detoxifying the body in cancer patients is a powerful and effective way to support your body's natural healing processes. By incorporating ingredients like turmeric, ginger, and oranges into your juicing routine, you can create delicious and nutritious juices that will help reduce inflammation, detoxify your body, and boost your overall health. Give this Anti-Inflammatory Turmeric Juice recipe a try and experience the benefits for yourself.

Immune-Boosting Ginger Shot

In the world of juicing for detoxifying the body in cancer patients, the immune-boosting ginger shot is a powerful weapon. Ginger, known for its anti-inflammatory properties, has been used for centuries in traditional medicine to boost the immune system and fight off illness. By incorporating ginger into a daily juicing routine, cancer patients can support their body's natural defenses and improve overall health.

To make an immune-boosting ginger shot, simply combine fresh ginger root with a splash of lemon juice and a pinch of cayenne pepper. Ginger is rich in antioxidants and contains compounds that have been shown to reduce inflammation and support the immune system. Lemon juice adds a burst of vitamin C, which is essential for immune function, while cayenne pepper provides a kick of heat that can help to stimulate circulation and improve digestion.

Drinking a ginger shot each day can help to detoxify the body and boost the immune system, making it an essential addition to any cancer-fighting juicing routine. By supporting the body's natural defenses, ginger shots can help cancer patients to feel stronger and more resilient as they undergo treatment. The anti-inflammatory properties of ginger can also help to reduce pain and inflammation, making it a valuable tool in managing side effects of cancer treatment.

In addition to its immune-boosting properties, ginger is also known for its ability to aid digestion and reduce nausea. Cancer patients undergoing treatment often experience digestive issues and nausea as side effects, making ginger shots a valuable tool for managing these symptoms. By incorporating ginger shots into their daily routine, cancer patients can support their digestive health and reduce feelings of nausea, improving their overall quality of life during treatment.

Overall, the immune-boosting ginger shot is a powerful tool for cancer patients looking to detoxify their bodies and improve their health. By incorporating this simple and delicious shot into their daily routine, cancer patients can support their immune system, reduce inflammation, aid digestion, and manage symptoms like nausea. With its potent combination of ginger, lemon juice, and cayenne pepper, the ginger shot is a must-have for anyone looking to boost their health and fight cancer from within.

Cleansing Leafy Green Juice

Cleansing Leafy Green Juice is a powerful tool in the fight against cancer and can play a crucial role in detoxifying the body. Packed with essential vitamins, minerals, and antioxidants, leafy greens such as kale, spinach, and Swiss chard are known for their cancer-fighting properties. By incorporating these nutrient-dense ingredients into your daily juicing routine, you can support your body's natural detoxification processes and boost your overall health.

One of the key benefits of Cleansing Leafy Green Juice is its ability to alkalize the body. Cancer thrives in an acidic environment, so by consuming alkaline-rich foods like leafy greens, you can create a more hostile environment for cancer cells to grow. Additionally, the high fiber content in leafy greens can aid in the elimination of toxins from the body, further supporting the detoxification process.

To make your own Cleansing Leafy Green Juice, simply combine a variety of leafy greens with other detoxifying ingredients such as cucumber, celery, and lemon in a juicer. Experiment with different combinations to find a flavor that you enjoy and be sure to drink your juice immediately to maximize its nutritional benefits. Consuming Cleansing Leafy Green Juice on a regular basis can help to cleanse your body of harmful toxins and promote overall wellness.

In addition to juicing, it is important to maintain a healthy lifestyle by eating a balanced diet, staying hydrated, and getting regular exercise. By incorporating Cleansing Leafy Green Juice into your daily routine, you can give your body the support it needs to detoxify and fight cancer. Remember that juicing is just one component of a comprehensive approach to cancer prevention and treatment, so be sure to consult with a healthcare professional for personalized advice.

Overall, Cleansing Leafy Green Juice is a delicious and convenient way to boost your health and support your body's natural detoxification processes. By incorporating this nutrient-rich beverage into your daily routine, you can take an active role in fighting cancer and promoting overall wellness. So grab your juicer and start juicing your way to a healthier, cancer-free future.

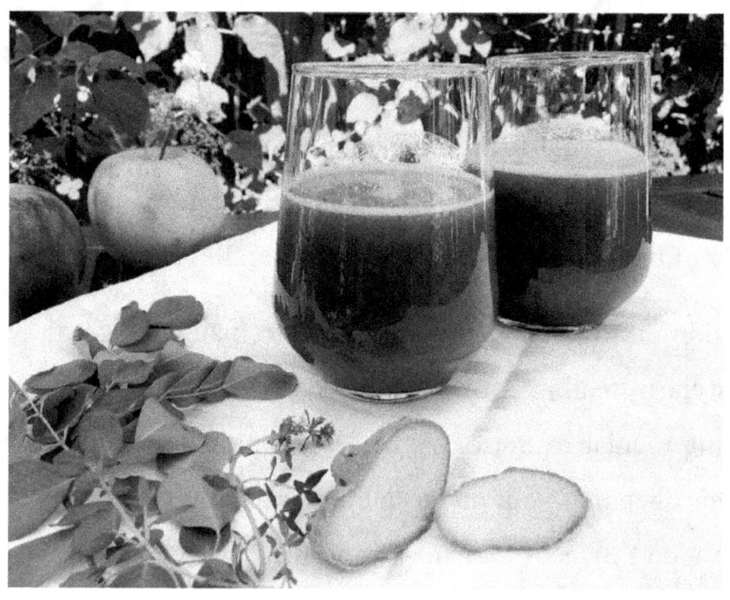

Chapter 4: Creating a Juicing Routine for Cancer Patients

Tips for Purchasing and Preparing Produce

When it comes to juicing for detoxifying the body in cancer patients, purchasing and preparing fresh produce is crucial. Here are some tips to help you make the most out of your juicing experience:

1. Buy organic whenever possible: Organic produce is free from harmful pesticides and chemicals that can further burden the body's detoxification systems. Look for the USDA organic label to ensure that you are getting the highest quality fruits and vegetables for your juices.

2. Choose a variety of colors: Different colored fruits and vegetables contain different antioxidants and phytochemicals that can help support the body's detoxification processes. Try to include a rainbow of colors in your juice recipes to ensure you are getting a wide range of nutrients.

3. Wash produce thoroughly: Even if you are buying organic produce, it is important to wash fruits and vegetables thoroughly before juicing to remove any dirt, bacteria, or residue. Use a produce brush or a mixture of water and vinegar to clean your produce before juicing.

4. Use a high-quality juicer: Investing in a high-quality juicer can make a big difference in the quality of your juices. Look for a juicer that is easy to clean, efficient at extracting juice, and has a variety of settings to accommodate different types of produce.

5. Juice in small batches: Freshly made juice is most beneficial when consumed immediately, as it can quickly lose its nutrient content and freshness. Try to juice in small batches and drink your juice right away to maximize its health benefits.

By following these tips for purchasing and preparing produce for your cancer-fighting juicing journey, you can ensure that you are getting the most out of your detoxification efforts. Remember to listen to your body and consult with a healthcare provider before making any significant changes to your diet, especially if you are undergoing cancer treatment.

Incorporating Juicing into Your Daily Routine

Incorporating juicing into your daily routine can be a powerful tool in detoxifying your body and boosting your overall health, especially for cancer patients. Juicing provides a concentrated source of essential nutrients, vitamins, and antioxidants that can help support your body's natural detoxification processes and strengthen your immune system. By incorporating juicing into your daily routine, you can give your body the extra support it needs to fight off cancer cells and promote overall wellness.

One of the easiest ways to incorporate juicing into your daily routine is to start your day with a fresh juice. By replacing your usual breakfast with a nutrient-rich juice, you can kickstart your metabolism and flood your body with essential vitamins and minerals. Try experimenting with different combinations of fruits and vegetables to find a mix that you enjoy and that provides maximum health benefits. For cancer patients, incorporating anti-inflammatory ingredients such as turmeric, ginger, and leafy greens can be particularly beneficial.

Another way to incorporate juicing into your daily routine is to have a juice as a mid-morning or afternoon snack. Instead of reaching for processed snacks or sugary treats, opt for a freshly made juice to give your body a natural energy boost and keep your cravings in check. Juicing can also be a great way to hydrate your body, especially for cancer patients undergoing treatment that can be dehydrating. Keeping your body well-hydrated is essential for supporting your body's detoxification processes and promoting overall health.

In addition to incorporating juicing into your daily routine, it's important to pair your juices with a balanced diet rich in whole foods. While juicing can provide a concentrated source of nutrients, it's important to also consume a variety of whole fruits, vegetables, lean proteins, and whole grains to ensure you're getting all the essential nutrients your body needs. By combining juicing with a healthy diet and regular exercise, you can create a comprehensive wellness plan that supports your body in fighting off cancer cells and promoting overall health.

Overall, incorporating juicing into your daily routine can be a simple yet effective way to detoxify your body and boost your health, especially for cancer patients. By starting your day with a fresh juice, enjoying a juice as a snack, and pairing your juices with a balanced diet, you can give your body the extra support it needs to fight off cancer cells and promote overall wellness. Juicing can be a delicious and convenient way to flood your body with essential nutrients and antioxidants, helping to strengthen your immune system and support your body's natural detoxification processes.

How to Listen to Your Body's Needs

Listening to your body's needs is crucial, especially when you are battling cancer. Your body has its way of communicating with you, and it is essential to pay attention to these signals to give it the care and nourishment it requires. One way to tune in to your body's needs is through juicing. Juicing can help detoxify your body and boost your health, providing it with essential nutrients that support your immune system and aid in the fight against cancer.

When it comes to juicing for detoxifying the body in cancer patients, it is important to listen to what your body is telling you. If you are feeling fatigued, your body may be in need of more energy-boosting ingredients like leafy greens and citrus fruits. If you are experiencing digestive issues, incorporating ingredients like ginger and mint can help soothe your stomach and aid in digestion. By listening to your body's signals, you can tailor your juicing recipes to meet your specific needs and promote healing from within.

Another way to listen to your body's needs is by paying attention to any cravings you may have. Cravings can often indicate deficiencies in certain nutrients, so it is essential to address these cravings with healthy, nutrient-rich ingredients in your juices. For example, if you are craving something sweet, try adding fruits like berries or apples to your juices. If you are craving something salty, consider adding ingredients like celery or cucumber to your recipes. By honoring your body's cravings with healthy alternatives, you can nourish your body and support its healing process.

In addition to listening to your body's needs through cravings, it is also essential to pay attention to how your body responds to different ingredients in your juices. Some people may have sensitivities or allergies to certain foods, so it is crucial to be mindful of how your body reacts after consuming a specific ingredient. If you notice any negative reactions such as bloating, digestive discomfort, or skin issues, it may be a sign that your body is not responding well to that ingredient. By listening to these signals, you can make adjustments to your juicing recipes to better suit your body's needs and promote overall well-being.

Overall, listening to your body's needs is a fundamental aspect of juicing for detoxifying the body in cancer patients. By tuning in to your body's signals, addressing cravings with healthy alternatives, and paying attention to how your body responds to different ingredients, you can tailor your juicing recipes to support your healing journey. Remember, your body knows best what it needs to thrive, so trust in its wisdom and nourish it with the nutrients it craves. By listening to your body and providing it with the care and nourishment it requires, you can boost your health, detoxify your body, and support your fight against cancer.

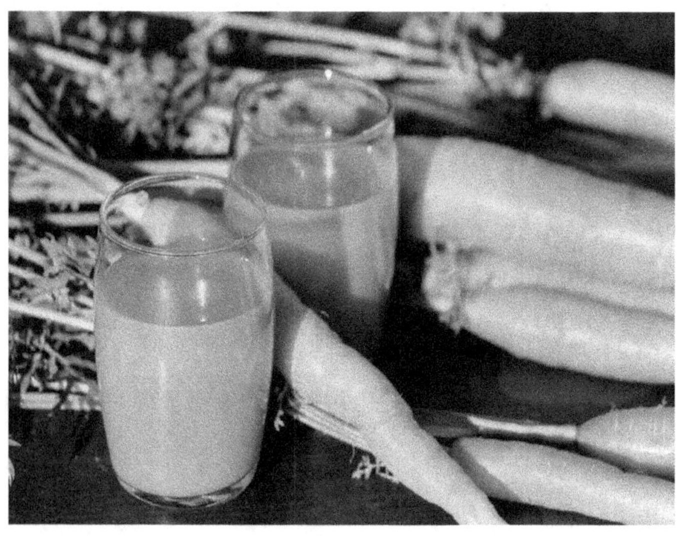

Chapter 5: Additional Lifestyle Changes for Cancer-Fighting Success

Incorporating Exercise into Your Routine

Incorporating exercise into your daily routine is essential for maintaining a healthy lifestyle, especially for cancer patients who are looking to detoxify their bodies and boost their health. Exercise not only helps improve physical strength and endurance but also plays a crucial role in reducing the risk of cancer recurrence and improving overall well-being. By combining regular exercise with a healthy juicing regimen, cancer patients can maximize the benefits of their treatment and enhance their body's ability to fight off cancer cells.

One of the key benefits of incorporating exercise into your routine is that it helps to improve circulation and oxygen flow throughout the body. This is particularly important for cancer patients, as it can help to flush out toxins and waste products that may contribute to cancer growth. By engaging in regular aerobic exercise such as walking, jogging, or cycling, cancer patients can help to increase their body's ability to detoxify and cleanse itself, leading to improved overall health and well-being.

In addition to improving circulation, exercise also helps to boost the immune system and reduce inflammation in the body. This is important for cancer patients, as chronic inflammation has been linked to an increased risk of cancer and can hinder the body's ability to fight off cancer cells. By incorporating strength training exercises into your routine, cancer patients can help to strengthen their immune system and reduce inflammation, leading to a lower risk of cancer recurrence and improved overall health.

Furthermore, exercise plays a crucial role in reducing stress and anxiety, which are common side effects of cancer treatment. By engaging in activities such as yoga, Pilates, or tai chi, cancer patients can help to calm their mind and reduce stress levels, leading to improved mental health and a greater sense of well-being. In combination with a healthy juicing regimen, exercise can help cancer patients to detoxify their bodies and boost their health from the inside out.

Overall, incorporating exercise into your routine is essential for cancer patients looking to detoxify their bodies and boost their health. By combining regular aerobic exercise, strength training, and stress-reducing activities, cancer patients can improve circulation, boost their immune system, reduce inflammation, and reduce stress levels, leading to improved overall health and well-being. By making exercise a priority in your daily routine, you can maximize the benefits of your juicing regimen and enhance your body's ability to fight off cancer cells and improve your quality of life.

Stress Management Techniques

Stress can be a major factor in exacerbating the symptoms of cancer and can hinder the body's ability to heal. Therefore, it is crucial for cancer patients to learn and implement effective stress management techniques to support their overall well-being. In this subchapter, we will explore various strategies that can help individuals cope with stress and improve their quality of life during cancer treatment.

One powerful stress management technique is mindfulness meditation. This practice involves focusing on the present moment without judgment, allowing individuals to cultivate a sense of calm and inner peace. Research has shown that mindfulness meditation can reduce stress, anxiety, and depression in cancer patients, as well as improve overall emotional well-being. By incorporating meditation into their daily routine, cancer patients can better cope with the challenges of their diagnosis and treatment.

Another effective stress management technique is deep breathing exercises. Deep breathing can help activate the body's relaxation response, reducing the production of stress hormones and promoting a sense of calm. Cancer patients can practice deep breathing exercises throughout the day, especially during moments of heightened stress or anxiety. By taking slow, deep breaths and focusing on their inhalation and exhalation, individuals can create a sense of relaxation and ease in both the mind and body.

Physical activity is also a powerful tool for managing stress. Exercise has been shown to release endorphins, the body's natural feel-good chemicals, which can help reduce stress and improve mood. Cancer patients can engage in gentle forms of exercise, such as walking, yoga, or tai chi, to help alleviate stress and promote relaxation. By incorporating regular physical activity into their routine, individuals can boost their overall well-being and cope more effectively with the challenges of cancer treatment.

In addition to these techniques, maintaining a healthy diet and practicing self-care can also help individuals manage stress during cancer treatment. Eating a balanced diet rich in fruits, vegetables, and whole grains can provide the body with essential nutrients and support overall health. Engaging in activities that bring joy and relaxation, such as spending time with loved ones, reading, or listening to music, can also help individuals reduce stress and improve their emotional well-being. By incorporating these stress management techniques into their daily routine, cancer patients can better cope with the challenges of their diagnosis and treatment, ultimately supporting their overall health and well-being.

Importance of Sleep for Healing

In the world of cancer treatment, the importance of sleep for healing cannot be overstated. Sleep is essential for the body to repair and regenerate itself, especially during times of illness. When you are juicing to detoxify your body and boost your health, getting enough sleep is crucial to support your body's natural healing processes.

During sleep, the body goes into a state of rest and repair. This is when the immune system is most active, fighting off infections and repairing damaged cells. For cancer patients undergoing treatment, sleep is even more important as it can help the body recover from the harsh effects of chemotherapy and radiation therapy. Getting enough rest can also help reduce inflammation in the body, which is crucial for cancer patients looking to boost their overall health.

Lack of sleep can have detrimental effects on the body, especially for cancer patients. It can weaken the immune system, making it harder for the body to fight off infections and heal itself. Inadequate sleep can also lead to increased levels of stress hormones, which can further compromise the body's ability to heal. By prioritizing sleep as part of your juicing regimen, you can give your body the rest it needs to support its natural healing processes.

In addition to benefiting the body physically, sleep also plays a crucial role in mental and emotional well-being. Cancer patients often experience high levels of stress and anxiety, which can impact their ability to heal. Getting enough sleep can help regulate mood and improve mental clarity, making it easier to cope with the challenges of cancer treatment. By incorporating healthy sleep habits into your juicing routine, you can support your overall well-being and enhance the healing process.

In conclusion, the importance of sleep for healing cannot be understated, especially for cancer patients juicing to detoxify their bodies. By prioritizing rest and making sleep a priority, you can support your body's natural healing processes, boost your immune system, and improve your overall well-being.

Remember, a good night's sleep is just as important as a healthy diet and regular exercise when it comes to fighting cancer and promoting optimal health.

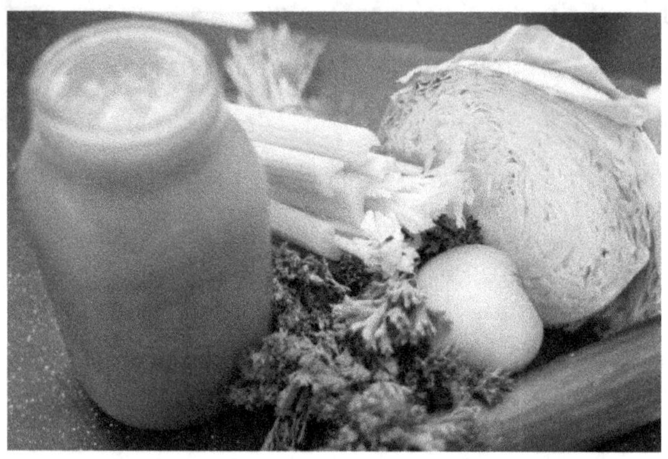

Chapter 6: Juicing for Long-Term Health and Prevention

Maintaining a Balanced Diet Post-Treatment

After undergoing cancer treatment, it is crucial for adults to focus on maintaining a balanced diet to support their overall health and well-being. Juicing can be a powerful tool in achieving this goal, as it provides a convenient and tasty way to incorporate a variety of nutrients into your daily routine. In this subchapter, we will discuss the importance of maintaining a balanced diet post-treatment and how juicing can play a key role in supporting your body's recovery.

One of the key benefits of juicing for detoxifying the body in cancer patients is that it allows you to easily consume a wide range of fruits and vegetables in a concentrated form.

This can be especially beneficial for individuals who may have difficulty eating large quantities of whole foods due to side effects from treatment. By juicing a combination of fruits and vegetables, you can ensure that your body receives the essential vitamins, minerals, and antioxidants it needs to support your immune system and promote healing.

When focusing on maintaining a balanced diet post-treatment, it is important to prioritize nutrient-dense foods that can help support your body's recovery. Juicing can be a convenient way to incorporate a variety of these foods into your diet, such as leafy greens, berries, and citrus fruits. These foods are rich in antioxidants, which can help protect your cells from damage and reduce inflammation in the body.

In addition to supporting your physical health, maintaining a balanced diet post-treatment can also help improve your mental and emotional well-being. Juicing can be a therapeutic practice that allows you to connect with your body and nourish yourself from the inside out. By taking the time to prepare and enjoy fresh juices, you can cultivate a sense of mindfulness and self-care that can be beneficial for your overall healing journey.

Overall, maintaining a balanced diet post-treatment is essential for supporting your body's recovery and promoting long-term health. Juicing can be a valuable tool in achieving this goal, as it provides a convenient and delicious way to incorporate a variety of essential nutrients into your daily routine. By prioritizing nutrient-dense foods and focusing on self-care through juicing, you can support your body's healing process and optimize your overall well-being as a cancer survivor.

Continuing to Detoxify Your Body

Now that you have started your journey towards detoxifying your body with juicing, it is important to continue with your efforts in order to achieve optimal results. Detoxification is a process that takes time and dedication, but the benefits are well worth the effort, especially for cancer patients. By continuing to detoxify your body through juicing, you can help to eliminate harmful toxins, boost your immune system, and improve your overall health and well-being.

One of the key components of continuing to detoxify your body is to incorporate a variety of fruits and vegetables into your juicing routine. Different fruits and vegetables contain different vitamins, minerals, and antioxidants that can help to cleanse and detoxify your body in different ways. By mixing and matching different fruits and vegetables in your juices, you can ensure that you are getting a wide range of nutrients that will help to support your body's natural detoxification processes.

In addition to juicing a variety of fruits and vegetables, it is also important to drink plenty of water throughout the day to help flush out toxins from your body. Water is essential for hydrating your cells and organs, and it can also help to support your body's natural detoxification processes. Aim to drink at least eight glasses of water a day, and consider adding lemon or cucumber slices to your water for added detoxification benefits.

Another important aspect of continuing to detoxify your body is to incorporate regular exercise into your routine. Exercise helps to stimulate your lymphatic system, which is responsible for eliminating toxins from your body. By engaging in regular physical activity, you can help to support your body's natural detoxification processes and improve your overall health and well-being.

In conclusion, continuing to detoxify your body through juicing is a powerful way to support your body's natural detoxification processes and improve your overall health and well-being. By incorporating a variety of fruits and vegetables into your juicing routine, drinking plenty of water, and engaging in regular exercise, you can help to eliminate harmful toxins, boost your immune system, and reduce your risk of cancer. Remember, detoxification is a journey, so be patient and consistent in your efforts, and you will soon reap the rewards of a healthier, cleaner body.

Preventing Cancer Recurrence with Juicing

Juicing has become a popular trend among adults looking to boost their health and detoxify their bodies. For cancer patients, juicing can be a powerful tool in preventing cancer recurrence. By incorporating a variety of fruits and vegetables into your daily juicing routine, you can provide your body with the essential nutrients it needs to fight off cancer cells and strengthen your immune system.

One of the key benefits of juicing for cancer prevention is the high concentration of antioxidants found in fruits and vegetables. Antioxidants help to neutralize harmful free radicals in the body that can lead to cancer development. By juicing a rainbow of colorful fruits and vegetables, you can ensure that you are getting a wide range of antioxidants to protect your cells from damage and reduce the risk of cancer recurrence.

In addition to antioxidants, juicing can also help to alkalize the body and reduce inflammation, both of which are key factors in preventing cancer growth. By including alkalizing ingredients such as leafy greens, cucumbers, and celery in your juices, you can create a more alkaline environment in your body that is less hospitable to cancer cells. Similarly, anti-inflammatory ingredients like turmeric, ginger, and berries can help to combat chronic inflammation, which has been linked to cancer development.

When juicing for cancer prevention, it is important to focus on organic, pesticide-free produce whenever possible. Pesticides and other toxins found in conventionally grown fruits and vegetables can actually contribute to cancer development, so opting for organic produce can help to reduce your exposure to these harmful chemicals.

Additionally, be sure to wash all produce thoroughly before juicing to remove any residual pesticides or contaminants.

Overall, juicing can be a powerful tool in preventing cancer recurrence by providing your body with essential nutrients, antioxidants, and anti-inflammatory compounds. By incorporating a variety of fruits and vegetables into your daily juicing routine, you can support your body's natural defenses against cancer and promote overall health and well-being. So grab your juicer and start juicing your way to a healthier, cancer-free future.

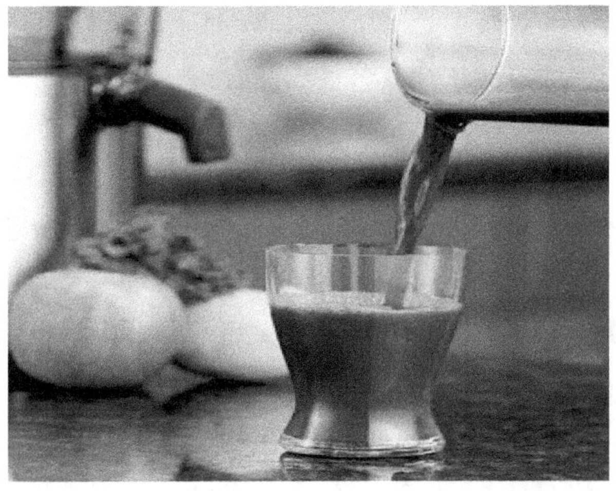

Chapter 7: Resources and Support for Cancer Patients

Finding Support Groups

When faced with a cancer diagnosis, it is important to remember that you are not alone. Support groups can provide a valuable source of emotional support, information, and encouragement during this challenging time. Finding the right support group can make a significant difference in your cancer journey.

One of the first steps in finding a support group is to ask your healthcare provider for recommendations. They may be able to connect you with local groups or online communities that cater to individuals going through a similar experience. Additionally, hospitals and cancer treatment centers often host support groups for patients and their families, providing a safe space to share experiences and learn from others.

Online resources can also be a helpful tool in finding support groups. Websites such as the American Cancer Society or Cancer Care offer directories of support groups based on cancer type, location, and specific needs. These online communities can provide a wealth of information and connections to others who are going through similar challenges.

It is important to find a support group that aligns with your personal preferences and needs. Some groups may focus on emotional support, while others may offer practical advice on managing treatment side effects or navigating the healthcare system. Consider attending a few different groups to find the one that feels like the best fit for you.

Remember that support groups are just one resource in your cancer-fighting journey. Juicing for detoxifying the body can also play a significant role in boosting your health and overall well-being. By combining the power of a supportive community with healthy lifestyle choices such as juicing, you can empower yourself to take control of your health and fight cancer with resilience and strength.

Working with a Nutritionist

Working with a nutritionist can be an invaluable resource for cancer patients looking to detoxify their bodies and boost their health through juicing. Nutritionists are experts in the field of food and nutrition, and can provide personalized guidance on how to optimize your juicing regimen for maximum health benefits. When working with a nutritionist, they will take into account your individual health needs, dietary preferences, and goals to create a customized juicing plan that is tailored to your specific needs.

One of the key benefits of working with a nutritionist is their ability to help you navigate the complex world of juicing and nutrition. They can help you understand the nutritional content of different fruits and vegetables, as well as how to combine them in a way that maximizes their health benefits. Additionally, a nutritionist can help you identify any potential nutrient deficiencies in your diet and recommend specific foods or supplements to address them.

Another important aspect of working with a nutritionist is their ability to provide ongoing support and accountability. By regularly meeting with a nutritionist, you can stay motivated and on track with your juicing goals. They can help you troubleshoot any challenges or setbacks you may encounter, and provide encouragement and guidance to help you stay focused on your health goals.

In addition to providing guidance on juicing and nutrition, a nutritionist can also help you make other lifestyle changes that can support your overall health and well-being. This may include recommendations for exercise, stress management techniques, and other strategies to improve your overall health and reduce your risk of cancer recurrence. By working with a nutritionist, you can take a comprehensive approach to your health that addresses the root causes of illness and promotes long-term wellness.

In conclusion, working with a nutritionist can be an important part of your journey to detoxify your body and boost your health through juicing. By providing personalized guidance, ongoing support, and expert advice, a nutritionist can help you optimize your juicing regimen and make positive changes to your overall health and well-being. If you are a cancer patient looking to incorporate juicing into your health routine, consider working with a nutritionist to help you achieve your health goals and improve your quality of life.

Accessing Additional Information and Research

When it comes to juicing for detoxifying the body in cancer patients, it is important to have access to reliable and up-to-date information and research. There are many resources available that can provide valuable insights into the benefits of juicing for cancer patients, as well as tips on how to incorporate juicing into a healthy lifestyle. One of the best ways to access this information is through reputable websites and online forums dedicated to cancer-fighting juicing.

In addition to online resources, there are also many books and publications that can provide valuable information on juicing for cancer patients. These resources often contain in-depth research and studies that support the benefits of juicing in detoxifying the body and boosting overall health. By exploring these resources, cancer patients can gain a better understanding of how juicing can play a role in their treatment and recovery journey.

Attending seminars, workshops, and conferences focused on juicing for cancer patients can also be a great way to access additional information and research. These events often feature experts in the field who can provide valuable insights and advice on how to incorporate juicing into a cancer-fighting regimen. By attending these events, cancer patients can interact with others who are on a similar journey and gain inspiration and motivation to continue their juicing efforts.

Another important way to access additional information and research on juicing for cancer patients is through speaking with healthcare professionals. Doctors, nutritionists, and other medical professionals can provide valuable guidance on how to incorporate juicing into a cancer treatment plan. By consulting with these experts, cancer patients can ensure that they are juicing in a safe and effective manner that complements their overall health and wellness goals.

In conclusion, accessing additional information and research on juicing for detoxifying the body in cancer patients is crucial for those looking to improve their health and well-being. By exploring online resources, books, attending events, and consulting with healthcare professionals, cancer patients can gain valuable insights into the benefits of juicing and how it can play a role in their cancer-fighting journey. With the right information and support, cancer patients can harness the power of juicing to detoxify their bodies and boost their overall health.

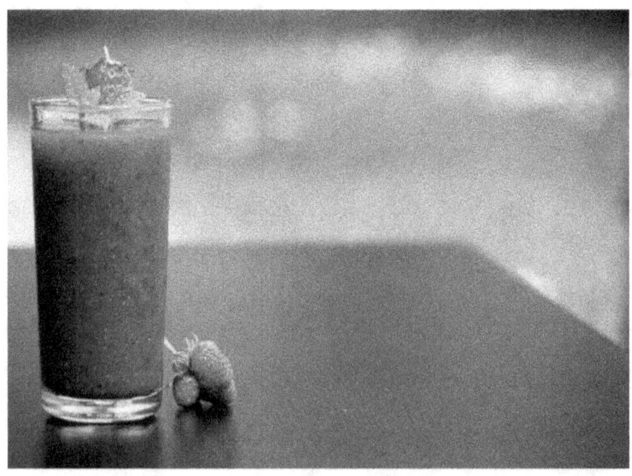

Chapter 8: Conclusion and Final Thoughts

Reflecting on Your Juicing Journey

As you reach the end of this juicing guide, take a moment to reflect on your juicing journey thus far. Whether you are just starting out or have been juicing for a while, it is important to acknowledge the progress you have made in improving your health and detoxifying your body. Juicing is not just about drinking delicious and nutritious juices; it is also about taking control of your health and making positive changes in your lifestyle.

Think back to when you first started juicing. What were your goals? Did you want to boost your immune system, improve your digestion, or detoxify your body? As you reflect on these goals, take note of how far you have come in achieving them. Have you noticed improvements in your energy levels, skin health, or overall well-being? Celebrate these victories and use them as motivation to continue on your juicing journey.

Consider the challenges you have faced along the way. Maybe you struggled to find the time to juice every day, or you found it difficult to stick to a juicing routine. Reflect on how you overcame these obstacles and what strategies worked best for you. Remember that setbacks are a normal part of any journey, and it is important to learn from them and move forward with a positive mindset.

Take a moment to think about the impact juicing has had on your life. Have you noticed any changes in your body, mind, or spirit since incorporating juicing into your daily routine? How has juicing helped you on your path to detoxifying your body and boosting your health? By reflecting on these questions, you can gain a deeper understanding of the power of juicing and its ability to transform your life.

As you continue on your juicing journey, remember to stay committed to your goals and prioritize your health. Keep experimenting with new recipes, ingredients, and techniques to keep things interesting and exciting. And most importantly, listen to your body and give it the nourishment it needs to thrive. By reflecting on your juicing journey and staying dedicated to your health and well-being, you can continue to detoxify your body and boost your overall health for years to come.

Celebrating Your Health Achievements

As you embark on your journey of juicing for detoxifying your body as a cancer patient, it is important to celebrate your health achievements along the way. Each step you take towards improving your health and well-being is a victory worth acknowledging and celebrating. Whether it's incorporating more nutrient-dense juices into your daily routine or making healthier food choices, every small change can have a significant impact on your overall health.

One way to celebrate your health achievements is by setting goals and tracking your progress. Start by identifying specific health goals that are important to you, such as increasing your energy levels, improving your digestion, or boosting your immune system. Then, track your progress by keeping a journal or using a health tracking app to monitor your symptoms, energy levels, and overall well-being. Celebrate each milestone you reach, whether it's drinking a certain amount of juice each day or sticking to a healthy meal plan for a week.

Another way to celebrate your health achievements is by treating yourself to something special. This could be a relaxing day at the spa, a new juicer or blender to make your favorite juices, or a healthy cooking class to learn new recipes and cooking techniques. By rewarding yourself for your hard work and dedication to your health, you are reinforcing positive habits and encouraging yourself to continue making healthy choices.

It's also important to celebrate your health achievements with others. Share your successes with friends and family members who support you on your journey to better health. Join a support group or online community of cancer patients who are also juicing for detoxification to share your experiences, tips, and success stories. By surrounding yourself with a supportive community, you can stay motivated and inspired to continue improving your health.

In conclusion, celebrating your health achievements is an important part of your journey to better health as a cancer patient juicing for detoxification. By setting goals, tracking your progress, treating yourself to rewards, and sharing your successes with others, you can stay motivated and inspired to continue making positive changes to your health and well-being. Remember to celebrate every small victory along the way, as each step you take towards better health is worth acknowledging and celebrating.

Looking Towards a Brighter, Healthier Future

In the journey towards fighting cancer, it is crucial to look towards a brighter, healthier future. Juicing has been proven to be an effective way to detoxify the body and boost overall health, making it a valuable tool in the fight against cancer. By incorporating fresh fruits and vegetables into your daily juicing routine, you can provide your body with the essential nutrients it needs to strengthen the immune system and promote healing.

Juicing for detoxification is especially important for cancer patients, as chemotherapy and other treatments can take a toll on the body. By juicing regularly, you can help rid your body of harmful toxins and free radicals, which can contribute to the growth and spread of cancer cells. Additionally, juicing can help improve digestion, reduce inflammation, and support the body's natural detoxification processes, all of which are essential for overall health and well-being.

When looking towards a brighter, healthier future, it is important to focus on incorporating a variety of fruits and vegetables into your juicing routine. Different fruits and vegetables contain unique compounds and nutrients that can help support the body in different ways. For example, cruciferous vegetables like broccoli and kale are known for their cancer-fighting properties, while berries are rich in antioxidants that can help protect cells from damage.

In addition to juicing for detoxification, it is also important to focus on other aspects of a healthy lifestyle, such as regular exercise, stress management, and adequate sleep. By taking a holistic approach to your health, you can support your body in its fight against cancer and promote overall well-being. Remember, every small step you take towards a healthier future can make a big difference in your journey towards better health and vitality.

In conclusion, looking towards a brighter, healthier future is essential for cancer patients who are juicing for detoxification. By incorporating a variety of fruits and vegetables into your juicing routine, focusing on overall health and well-being, and taking a holistic approach to your health, you can support your body in its fight against cancer and create a strong foundation for a healthier future. Remember, the choices you make today can have a lasting impact on your health and well-being tomorrow.